Run Your Ass Off!

The Ultimate Guide to Running for Rapid Weight Loss, Better Health and Injury Prevention

Max Fischwell

Please Leave Your Review of The Book At
www.amazon.com

ISBN-13: 978-1500347215

ISBN-10: 1500347213

First Printing, 2014

Printed in the United States of America

About the Author

Max Fischwell is about improving his life in various ways, and loves to share what he has accomplished by writing books so that his readers can learn to improve themselves as well.

One of his favorite past-times is to stay fit both physically and mentally. Therefore, one of his favorite endeavors that he has recently embarked upon is practicing yoga and meditation.

Max Fischwell loves yoga as it keeps you fit physically as well as mentally. However since meditation is an important aspect of yoga, Max Fischwell has taken a profound interest in studying meditation and loves practicing it, as it also has great benefits mentally by itself.

Right now Max Fischwell is in the process of maintaining his health from cardio and yoga and is always looking for ways he can educate and improve himself.

Table of Contents

Introduction

So there you are sitting on a bench or on your couch looking out of your window … and out of the blue one of "those runners" passes by. Running with their nice physique while you are sitting there wishing you could be just like them. So, what is stopping you? While you most certainly can come up with lame excuse after lame excuse, the real, definitive answer is simple: it's you.

It's true; you are the only thing stopping you from being one of those runners. Unless you have a physical handicap that prevents you from using your legs, then I can tell you right now you are more than capable of putting on a pair of sneakers and jogging around the block.

I mean, think about it. What else could be holding you back? It's certainly not money. That may be a reasonable excuse for not joining an expensive gym or fitness class. However, the beauty of running is that if you can afford a pair of sneakers and comfortable running clothes then you can afford to go running.

Now you might say that you don't have time. While I admit that this can be a challenge at times, think about this: do you think those other runners don't have busy lives as well? Do you think they just won the lottery and don't have a full-time job or kids to take care of?

So what is the difference between you and them? Well the answer comes down to dedication. At some point they made a conscious decision to make getting in shape a priority. Then they just did it. Let me make that point really clear. Instead of sitting on their asses and just thinking about it, they actually went out and did it.

So here is my challenge for you. Once you are done reading this book for the day, can you do me or better yet yourself this one small favor? Go out and run. It doesn't have to be for long.

Hell, it can just be around the block. The important thing is that you go out and do it. In fact if you are not in shape and can't even remember the last time you exercised I would advise you to take it slow.

Remember we all have to start somewhere. The important thing is to just start. I hope this book motivates you. I hope it helps give you the kick in the ass that we all sometimes need in life.

I also hope that you find this book informative and helpful in other ways as well. While running is pretty simple, once you start to make a habit of it, there are running techniques that will help you continue and grow your habit, as well as some challenges that you may encounter.

I will introduce you to the proper running form and how important your form is to prevent injuries. I will go over the most common injuries and the steps you can take to prevent them. I also will cover nutrition so you can get the most out of your running, as well as different types of running exercises to prevent boredom and build more muscle.

This is just some of what I will be covering in this information compact book. So on that note let's get started and talk about why you should consider running for weight loss anyway.

Top Five Reasons Why You Should Run to Lose Weight

If you are looking to slim down and lose extra body fat, research has shown that running may be the most effective way of shedding the pounds for an improved appearance. Instead of focusing on a strict diet plan that will leave you perpetually hungry and cause your body to go into starvation mode without key nutrients, it is more recommended that you lose fat through increased daily exercise.

While any exercise is good exercise for the body, it is hard to beat the results of running when it comes to losing weight. Whether you are a newbie or a seasoned runner, the following is an in-depth look at the top five perks of pavement pounding that make running the best exercise for weight loss.

1. More Burned Calories in Less Time

Although many mistakenly believe that running a mile and walking a mile can burn a similar number of calories, this myth holds no actual weight. Individuals who run are able to burn calories at a considerably faster rate than those walking or engaging in other low-intensity forms of exercise.

Since the number of calories burned while running is mostly determined by your body weight, you can typically expect to burn around 0.63 times your body weight on average per mile. For instance, an average 140-pound woman who runs at a 10-minute mile pace for an hour will be able to burn roughly 512 calories during her run. While this formula gives a good ballpark figure for determining how many calories you are torching, calorie burn can also be increased even further by running faster or longer with consistent practice.

Conveniently, running is also one of the most time-efficient exercises available because it enables runners to burn more calories in a considerably shorter time than walkers. After all, most people can run three or four times as far as they could walk in the same period of time. Even more importantly, running can be done alone, virtually anywhere, and there is no fancy expensive equipment needed beyond the basic running gear. Therefore, running is a quick, cost-effective, and accessible form of exercise that can burn many more calories in the long run.

2. Improved Muscle Tone and Physique

For those who have ever spent time watching a marathon race or visited the treadmills in a packed gym, chances are you are aware that runners often have the best bodies. Have you ever wondered why runners are able to maintain a toned figure, trim waistline, and enviable firm legs? Well, not only does running help to dramatically increase the amount of calories being torched in less the time, but it also helps shed body fat to uncover the lean toned muscle beneath. Along with noticing the digits on the scale dropping, running for weight loss also leads to reduced visible body fat, improved muscle tone, increased muscle size, and tightened cellulite for an enhanced physique.

When you are running, the primary muscles that are being used are your calves, hamstrings, quads, glutes, and core. As a result, it is no surprise that running is one of the most efficient methods of strengthening and toning your body while also blasting calories.

Although running often receives a bad reputation as a weight-bearing exercise for leading to chronic back pain, osteoarthritis, and even wrinkly skin, running actually builds stronger muscles and ligaments, especially in the hip and knee joints. These muscles can effectively protect various areas of the body from the cartilage decay that causes pain as well as inflammation with arthritis.

3. Decreased Risk for Major Health Concerns

Beyond simply gaining an amazing body and losing excess weight, taking up running can have even more important long-lasting effects that will put you on the right track to a longer, healthier life. Even if you only meet the minimum amount of physical activity recommended through running, science shows that your life expectancy will rise due to a significant reduction in major health risks.

Researchers at Stanford University's School of Medicine discovered that running dramatically slows the aging clock and that runners have a 39% lower risk of suffering an early death in comparison to other healthy adults of the same age. In fact, smokers can add 4.1 years to their life, cancer survivors can extend their life for 5.3 more years, and those with heart disease can gain up to 4.3 years by becoming a regular runner.

While everyone is aware that running helps build muscles and bones, nearly every other system in the human body receives health benefits as a direct result of running too. As running helps to reduce body fat and burn extra calories, the cardio exercise can help the occurrence of heart disease, type 2 diabetes, metabolic syndrome, osteoporosis, Alzheimer's disease, and even cancer!

While running may not be the overall cure for cancer, research has shown that hitting the pavement or the treadmill can be an excellent way to reduce your chances of developing many kinds of cancer. Furthermore, if you have already have been diagnosed with certain forms of cancer, running can help to improve your overall quality of life while undergoing the painstaking process of chemotherapy treatments.

4. Enhanced Mental Health: Runner's High

As with any other type of exercise for losing weight, if you do not truly enjoy it, chances are pretty high that you will not stick with it for a long period of time. Along with giving you a physical edge for shedding unwanted pounds for a leaner look, running has been proven to dramatically improve mental health.

With just 30 minutes of running during one week, you could boost your mood, enhance your concentration, and even improve the quality of your sleep. Running is also an extraordinary stress reliever that enables runners to fall into a rhythm that can quickly lull the mind into a meditative state where worries simply fall away. Instead of reaching for comfort foods, going for a run will be able to take you to a "stress-free" zone where just you, your body, and the environment around you exist.

Many runners also happily report that they experience what has been termed a "runner's high" before and after hitting the pavement. No matter how good or bad you may feel at a certain moment, running is able to make you feel better through an instant rush of feel-good hormones to your brain. Scientists have discovered that moderate to intense running triggers the release of cocaine-like brain chemicals known as endocannabinoids.

In addition, the areas in the brain that are closely linked with mood changes are flooded with endorphins for happy sensations during a run. Therefore, many runners indicate that the euphoria makes them want to go for another run and stick to an exercise schedule that is conducive to weight loss.

5. Increased Metabolic Rate

Since it takes a large amount of effort to move your entire body weight at a rapid speed without assistance, running is an effective method of improving your metabolic rate to burn extra calories even when you are sedentary or at rest. Running is able to stimulate more "after burn" in our bodies well after completing the workout than low-intensity exercises, such as walking and swimming. When two individuals run and walk the same exact distance, health experts indicate that the runner will lose far more weight than the walker.

This is most likely to happen due to the fact that running enables your resting energy expenditure to maintain its elevated state after the run. Accordingly, it is not surprising that a study in the Journal of Medicine and Science in Sports and Exercise found that runners lost 90% more weight than those who walked.

Overall, several studies have proven that running is a more effective method for shedding extra pounds and burning calories than other forms of exercise, especially walking. While running is a great way to improve fitness as well as achieve substantial weight loss, it is important to remember that running must be accompanied by a balanced diet to have the best results. In order to ensure you are on the right track to a sound running program and are eating enough calories to fuel your workouts, it is recommended that you consult with a nutritionist or other healthcare professional to make sure you maximize the weight loss achieved through running.

Running Gear

Essential Basic Running Gear for Beginners

Although running is highly regarded as being the most effective method of exercise for burning calories and shedding extra weight, it is also considered one of the simplest sports available with very little specialized equipment needed. Instead of wasting money buying a closet full of new gear, the general rule of thumb when it comes to running is "quality over quantity."

However, since it is extremely important that you feel comfortable in what you are wearing and have suitable clothing for the exercise, there are a few running gear staples that are well worth the investment. If you are a newbie to running, the following are the most basic essentials in running gear for a cool, comfortable workout no matter how far you go.

Your Most Important Gear: Running Shoes

In order to ensure that your body has the protection and support it
needs during your run, you are going to need a good pair of running
shoes that are specifically designed for running. Rather than pulling
out tennis shoes or digging up an old beat-up pair of running shoes
from the bottom of your closet, it is recommended that you invest in
purchasing a brand-new fresh pair of running shoes.

While the running shoes do not need to be expensive nor do they have
to be outfitted with all of the latest bells and whistles, it is essential
that you do not short-change yourself by underestimating the
tremendous power of having a decent running shoe. After all, wearing
improper running shoes is often the most prominent cause of running
injuries.

Therefore, it is best to take a trip to your local sports store to find well-
cushioned shoes that have been manufactured to provide the comfort
needed when running. With the help of an expert, you will be able to
evaluate your, gait, and running style to find the ideal shoes that match
your individualized running needs.

When you go shopping for your new pair of shoes, it is smart to go in
the afternoon after lunchtime because it is common for your feet to
expand throughout the day and you do not want a snug fit that will
cause blisters. As a beginner, your legs and feet will need all the

protection they can get from proper running shoes to prevent the occurrence of injury, which will certainly curb your enthusiasm for the sport.

What Clothes to Wear While Running

When you first endeavor into a running program, you will not necessarily have to rush out to find a whole new wardrobe filled with fancy clothing designed for running. If you have already been following an exercise plan, you can start out by wearing the comfortable clothing that you usually use to workout in.

However, there are some helpful tactics in dressing for running that you should be aware of. First and foremost, be sure you do not overdress and take into consideration that your body temperature will naturally rise quickly when running. For instance, if the temperature outside is above 60°F, you will likely only need to wear a shirt and shorts as your extra body heat will automatically add at least 15 degrees.

As you start becoming a more seasoned runner, you may want to try out more technical running clothing that will help wick away excess moisture to keep you cool as a cucumber during long runs. In any sports store, you will be able to find lightweight short and long sleeve t-shirts, tights, shorts, and waterproof jackets that enable more circulation through the fabric thanks to technological advancements.

Instead of cotton apparel that is often associated with irritation, look for clothing that is made from more technical materials, including nylon, lycra, and wool. While you want to remain comfortable during your run, also remember to wear reasonably tight, fight-hugging clothing to prevent the fabric from flapping and causing chafing.

Added Accessories for Runs

When you are just starting out, your basic running gear will simply include a great pair of running shoes designed to your feet style and comfortable breathable clothing. That being said, there are also some added accessories that could make you infinitely more comfortable during your running workouts as you go.

For the ladies, it is recommended that you wear a snug sports bra that provides sufficient support for running, but still allows air to circulation. Rather than wearing your everyday underwire bra, make sure you choose a sports bra that fits snugly under the bust, has wider straps that will not dig in, provides adequate coverage on the sides without any bulges, and wicks away the sweat that tends to accumulate in the region.

Not only is it important to have solid running shoes, but it is also recommended that you choose the right pair of socks that will keep your feet comfortable inside of them. While simple white sports socks will do, some runners prefer purchasing more technical socks made from wool or other synthetic fibers to absorb any moisture.

Furthermore, you may be interested in finding more advanced running socks that have been purposefully designed to add more padding in certain areas of the foot for enhanced support. Regardless, ensure that your socks will leave your feet comfortable so that you do not consequently slip and develop blisters.

If you are planning to run in the wee hours before sunrise or late at night after the sun has gone down, it is also crucial that you take additional safety precautions with specialized running gear. When you are running in the dark, you will want to guarantee that others on the road can see you and that you can see them as well.

Therefore, runners are typically encouraged to bring along a bright handheld LED light or wear a headlamp to alert drivers of their presence. For those who want to be absolutely sure that others will sense their movements, you may also want to consider wearing a reflective vest while running.

As technology continues to advance on a seemingly daily basis, there are also dozens of other gadgets on the market, ranging from the simple to the extremely sophisticated. You may want to invest in a GPS watch that will alert you to how fast you are running, your current heart rate level, your pace, and how far you have gone. In fact, the next section will delve further into heart rate monitors and the benefits of targeting certain heart rate zones with them.

Although some runners swear by certain running devices that provide instant feedback on fitness levels, others get by just fine without them. At the very least, your running gear will need to include a good pair of shoes and comfortable well-fitted clothing, but any other accessories are completely up to your own personal preferences.

Heart Rate Zones

Running With a Heart Rate Monitor

How can you determine whether you are putting in the right amount of effort needed to maximize your strength training and weight loss potential during every run? While many seasoned runners are able to simply perceive the intensity of their workout based on their breathing and pulse, others depend on some assistance in the form of a heart rate monitor.

Heart rate monitors can be extremely beneficial tools in training because they enable runners to read their pulse rate through a sensor that is conveniently placed on a chest strap. Most beginners are able to get by just fine by simply observing their exhaustion level and slowly down when getting tired on their own.

However once you start implementing more extreme running exercises like adding in sprint intervals or running more long distances such as a 10k or half or full marathon, you may want to consider investing in a heart rate monitor to get the most out of your running. If you are contemplating whether a heart rate monitor is right for you, read on to learn more about its benefits and how you can effectively implement training with heart rate zones.

Importance of Using a Heart Rate Monitor

When utilized in a proper fashion, heart rate monitors are valuable training tools that can serve as an indicator of your exercise intensity level while running based on your pulse rate. Since novice and even intermediate runners commonly make the mistake of not varying their intensity effectively to maximize results, a heart rate monitor is a helpful guide to precisely control the intensity of your workout. Not only will measuring your heart rate ensure that your body is working hard enough to burn enough calories and build muscle mass, but it is also essential for avoiding the overexertion that can lead to common running injuries.

In order to better understand your body's response to your workouts, it is recommended that you consider training with a heart rate monitor to hit specific zones for realizing your optimal potential. When working out with a heart rate monitor strapped to your chest, you will want to hit zones by falling into a specific percentage of your heart rate during each run. Due to the fact that running too fast can increase your danger for both burnout and injury, runners are typically encouraged to keep their heart rate in Zone 1 or 2 throughout the majority of their workouts.

Zone 1: Active Recovery

As the heart rate zone that is normally used as a warm-up or cool-down for each run, Zone 1 is referred to as Active Recovery because it involves running at a very comfortable pace without much effort. At 60 to 70% of the heart rate reserve, Zone 1 generally consists of a heart rate ranging between 139 and 152 beats per minute in easy or recovery runs. While it may seem counterintuitive, training in this zone can be highly effective for improving the heart's ability to pump blood as well as the muscles' capacity for utilizing oxygen. As a result, your body will become more efficient at feeding its muscles and metabolizing fat in energy production.

Zone 2: Aerobic Threshold

At 70 to 80% of the heart rate reserve, Zone 2 is the most common heart rate zone for training because it is the most efficient at helping the body to improve its overall cardiovascular health during runs. Also referred to as the Aerobic Threshold due to its comfortable pace that delivers a strong workout without interrupting the ability to have a conversation, Zone 2 is generally around 152 to 166 beats per minute. Not only does this heart rate zone help increase your body's overall muscular strength, but it also improves your cardio-respiratory system so that oxygen can be delivered to muscles and carbon dioxide eliminated. This is the zone you would want to be in typically when you are going for a longer than usual run.

Zone 3: Anaerobic Threshold

Generally occurring at around 80 to 90% of the heart rate reserve, Zone 3 is often called the Anaerobic Threshold or Lactate Threshold because it is the point at which the human body no longer is able to effectively remove lactic acid as rapidly as it is manufactured. While this pace should still be comfortable, it is hard enough that most runners will only be able to speak in a few short phrases while maintaining this heart rate zone of around 166 to 179 beats per minute. When running to achieve Zone 3, you will notice that your muscles will become fatigued and your breathing will be labored, but training within this zone will be beneficial for increasing your lactate threshold to enhance your overall running performance in your workouts. This is the zone you would want to be in when going for a tempo run, which I will delve into further at a later section.

Zone 4: V02 Max "Red Line" Zone

As you might expect from its name, the V02 Max "Red Line" Zone is the maximum heart rate zone that should be achieved while running. Since it consists of 90 to 100% of your total heart rate reserve, Zone 4 should only be attempted for very short periods of time by experienced runners who are extremely physically fit.

At around 179 to 192 beats per minute, Zone 4 involves hard effort at a sustainable pace in which conversation is very difficult. For the majority of runners, the V02 Max "Red Line" Zone is often reached at a 5K pace. Although training in this zone should be minimal, it can be helpful for enhancing your body's fast twitch muscle fibers and increasing your overall running speed.

How to Calculate Your Heart Rate Zones

Of course, the first step towards heart zone training is calculating your maximum heart rate. While runners have used the simple equation of 220 minus your age for several decades, researchers indicate that is may actually be up to 10 beats off for most of the general population. If you are comfortable using this method than that this is fine. However, if you want to be more exact you may want to find your V02 max heart rate by completing what is known as the Rockport Fitness Walking Test.

Start by walking at a fast sustainable pace for one mile with a heart rate monitor and then immediately record your maximum heart rate. Next, plug your data into the equation VO2 max = 132.853 - (0.0769 x Weight) - (0.3877 x Age) + (6.315 x Gender) - (3.2649 x Time) - (0.1565 x Heart beats in 10 seconds). For the gender portion of the formula, enter 1 if you are a male and 0 if you are a female. Since this is quite intensive, you can also conveniently use a V02 max heart rate calculator found online to do the math for you.

Once you have gathered data on your maximum heart rate for the V02 Max "Red Line" Zone, you will want to obtain your resting heart rate. In most cases, your resting heart rate can be best discovered by taking your pulse at your neck for a full minute as soon as you open your eyes in the morning, but before you step out of bed.

Next, you can calculate your heart rate reserve by taking your maximum heart rate and subtracting the resting heart rate. In order to know which numbers to target in each of the zones, multiply the heart rate reserve by the zone percentage in decimal form and then add back in the resting heart rate.

For example let's say your maximum heart rate is 180 and your resting heart rate is 70. You would then subtract the two to come up with your heart rate reserve at 110. Now let's say you want to run at the aerobic threshold at 70%. You would then take 110 x .70 to come up with 77. Now you would add 70 to come up with a target number of 147.

Overall, heart rate is one of the best indicators available for estimating your running intensity to target your workouts for optimal results. Since your heart rate as well as your thresholds will change continuously as you become more physically fit, you will need to repeatedly test your heart rate to ensure you are using accurate zones.

Although a heart rate monitor is a great tool for running, remember to not become a slave to it. As you become more experienced with running, you will notice that you can instead monitor the intensity of your workouts by perceived exertion and pace to realize your maximum potential as a runner.

Proper running form

How to Run with Proper Form

In order to achieve the best weight loss and fitness results, it is imperative that you run efficiently with a proper relaxed form. When you maintain an ideal body position, you are able to run with good form, use less energy, run faster, and avoid injury.

If you are noticing any tension in your arms, back, shoulders, neck, or hips, you most likely need to evaluate your running form and make some important adjustments. Therefore, read on to learn more about how you can recognize any inefficiencies, easily correct faulty habits, and practice proper running form from head to foot to get the most out of your workout safely and enjoyably.

Head

Whether you are running, walking, or doing any other daily activity, how you hold your head is one of the major factors that has an influence on your overall posture. Since your head position specifically dictates how efficiently you will be able to run, you must make sure that you look ahead naturally.

Instead of peering down at your feet or sightseeing along your path, face forward to let your eyes guide you. Be sure to keep your neck and back straightened, bring your shoulders into alignment, and avoid jutting your chin forward.

Shoulders/Neck

One of the most essential components of achieving a proper running form is maintaining a good, relaxed posture. As you might expect, the shoulders and neck play a crucial role in ensuring that the upper portion of your body remains relaxed and free of tension while running.

Instead of allowing your shoulders to ride high and your neck muscles to tighten in distress, you must make sure your shoulders stay low and loose in a natural leveled posture throughout the run. Since it is human nature for the neck to start hunching as you become more tired, take the time to shake your shoulders loose to release this built-up tension effectively.

Arms

Although running is primarily classified as an intensive lower-body exercise, you should never underestimate the power that your arms have on your running form. When our bodies begin to feel the effects of fatigue, we tend to make the common mistake of pulling the arms up close to the body in what is often termed the "chicken wing."

Whenever your arms are held tightly towards the side of your body, the result will be a shorter arm swing, shorter stride, and a slower pace. Your arms should be swinging mostly forward and back at the side of your body, with your elbows bent at a 90° angle at waist level.

Moving down from the arms, you must also be aware of your hands while running to ensure a proper form. Since your hands are responsible for having complete control over the tension that is experienced throughout your upper body, it is critical that you avoid clenching your fists at all costs.

While running, imagine yourself carrying a fragile egg each in each hand and allow your fingers to lightly touch your palm without crushing the egg. Whenever you feel your hands begin to clench, do not be afraid to let your arms drop for a few seconds to shake out the tension.

Chest/Torso

In order to realize the most optimal stride length and increase your
lung capacity to take more vital oxygen into your body, it is essential
that you keep your chest and torso straightened. Often referred to as
"running tall" by the world's most accomplished runners, the ideal
torso positioning involves allowing yourself to stretch upright to your
full height and keeping your back comfortably straight. While it may
be hard to avoid slouching as fatigue starts to set in, taking a deep
calming breath and exhaling slowly will help you naturally straighten
to the proper form.

Hips

Due to the fact that the hips are naturally the body's center of gravity,
maintaining the proper positioning of your hips is a major key towards
achieving good running posture. If your abdomen is straight, your hips
will automatically fall into the accurate alignment to point straight
ahead.

Since allowing your pelvis to tilt forward will increase the amount of
pressure being placed on your lower back and increase the risk of
injury, be sure to keep an upright torso and hips. For achieving the
desired position of your hips, you may want to imagine your pelvis is a
bowl filled with soup and consciously avoid tilting the bowl to spill the
soup.

Legs

While it may seem that running with a longer stride will translate into a faster finish time, it is important that runners avoid increasing their stride length by extending their feet too far forward in front of their body. Instead of over striding to run faster further like a sprinter, a proper running form for distance runners consists of a slight knee life, short stride, and a quick leg turnover drawn from the hips. With all of these elements combined together, your movement will stop diverting energy and begin facilitating more movements that are fluid.

When running with the appropriate stride length, your feet will land directly underneath your body without an extension, your knee will be slightly flexed for a natural bend on impact, and your shin will remain vertical as your foot lightly strikes the ground. If you notice your calf is extended forward in front of your body, decrease your stride length. Most running experts agree that around 180 steps each minute is the optimal tempo for achieving a proper running stride.

Feet

As you might expect, running properly will require you to have complete control over your ankles to ensure your feet are pushing off the ground with the force needed to propel you towards your goals. With each step, your feet should be hitting the ground lightly, touching the sole of your shoe between heel and mid-foot, and rapidly springing forward. In order to create the optimal level of force for pushing off the pavement, keep your ankles flexed, allow your calf muscles to propel you forward, and maintain a quiet, springy step for good running form.

Different Running Exercises

Eight Different Running Exercises to Spice Up Your Workout

If you find yourself becoming bored with your workouts or have reached a plateau in your weight loss, then it may be the perfect time to start changing things up with some different running exercises to prevent burnout from setting in. While running at the same speed everyday will still burn calories, you will need to increase your speed or resistance levels to really maximize your exercise potential.

Not only will mixing up your runs create more interest, but it will also help build muscle mass for more efficient weight loss. Building more muscle mass is essential for increasing your metabolic rate to burn even more calories when at rest, as well as strengthen the body's connective tissues to reduce the risk of injury. The following are some of the different types of runs that you may want to spice up your running schedule with for optimal results.

1. Tempo Runs

As one of the most common types of running exercises that is often a staple in many intermediate and advanced runners' programs, tempo runs are also referred to as lactate-threshold runs because they are effective at helping you develop your anaerobic threshold and increase your overall running speed. Basically, a tempo run involves running at a sustained and controlled pace that is considered a steady effort, rather than a fast race pace. Tempo runs are able to train your body to eliminate the built up lactate in your muscles more efficiently and rapidly, which also helps to prevent muscle fatigue.

In order to add a tempo run into your workout, you will want to warm up with five to ten minutes of slower running. Then, increase your pace gradually with peak speed coming about two-thirds into the workout for another 15 to 20 minutes for steady, hard and controlled running. As a general rule of thumb, make sure that you are pace yourself by your breathing.

For instance, if you are making more than two footfalls on an inhale and one footfall on an exhale, then you must slow down a little to reach this pace.

When doing a tempo run you are running about 85 – 90% of your maximum heart rate. What this essentially means is that you are running at a moderately difficult pace. If you find that you are able to carry on a conversation without any effort then you are probably going too slow and would need to pick up the pace a bit. You shouldn't be able to say more than a few words without any effort. After running at this pace for 15 – 20 minutes it is vital that you cool down by finishing the run workout with five to ten minutes at a slower jog pace.

2. The Fartlek

Whether you do regular jobs or tempo runs at some point you may find yourself reaching a plateau. You may think the only way to increase your aerobic system is to simply run longer. While this is certainly one option there is also another option as well. That of course is to increase your intensity. Of course the idea of running near top speed for your whole run is more than likely not a very viable option for you unless you perhaps significantly cut back on your distance. However, if you are looking to increase your intensity without cutting back on how far you run, than you may want to strongly consider running fartleks.

While this name may sound funny to us it actually translates to "speed play" in Swedish. The fartlek is often given the good reputation for being one of the best starter workouts for novices interested in testing the waters of speed and/or interval training. Fartleks involve running at an easy pace with different bursts of speed throughout the run at varying times, which can range anywhere from 15 seconds to three minutes.

Despite the funny name and the informality of this speed workout, fartlek exercises are excellent for building muscle mass as well as training your legs to absorb a multitude of paces and distances to become a better runner. Also the frequent sprinting bursts, helps you burn more calories making this ideal if you are trying to lose weight. This is because sprinting helps builds more lean muscles which overtime increases your metabolism.

Instead of hitting a boring track, fartlek workouts should be taken on a usual course on the road or trail so that there are plenty of random landmarks that you can choose from. After warming up for at least five to ten minutes, start a series of mixed intervals and recovery periods at your own preference. Since it is a variable exercise, you may wish to do shorter sprint intervals or longer intervals.

It is usually recommended that you choose a landmark, run hard to reach it, jog to recover, and then choose another landmark to repeat the process for as long as you want. As you practice fartlek exercises more frequently, you will be able to increase interval times as you become stronger and faster.

Running fartleks are ideal for the runner that is looking to get more out of their running workout without putting more time. Many of us are busy individuals and we just may not have the time to significantly increase our running volume. This is why fartleks can be a viable solution. You will get more benefit from your workout from the added sprints, and you won't need to increase the amount of time you go for a run. Not to mention fartleks can add a lot of variety to your running routine preventing you from getting bored. This of course is just another great benefit of running fartleks.

3. Long Runs

For those who are training to run a 10K, half marathon, or full marathon, long runs will eventually need to become your best friend and a staple of your training program. As you might expect from the name, long runs basically consist of extending how long you run once each week to push yourself for longer distances than you are accustomed to.

In most cases, runners will choose to do their long runs on a weekend and typically on the same day of week that the goal race will be falling on. While runners training for a marathon will usually do long runs for 16 miles or more, those preparing for a short run like a 5K may add long runs of over 3.1 miles.

If you are considering adding long runs to your program for added distance, it is recommended that you try to start by adding 10% to your longest run in recent training to ensure you are not pushing yourself too hard out of the gate. For example, if your longest distance recently was three miles, you may want to try running 3.3 miles the first week and 3.6 miles the second.

However, it is important to remember to cut back on your long runs once a month to give your muscles a chance to recover and maximize your endurance. Whenever you do a long run, be sure to slow your pace down a little so that you can achieve a steady run at an easy speed.

4. Hill Repeats

Once you have built up some stamina and endurance, hills are a natural way to add strength into your running schedule to more effectively build strong muscle mass. Since you must fight the natural effects of gravity to lift your entire body weight with your legs when running up an incline, hills are often compared to lifting weights for runners.

In fact running uphill can be one of the best workouts you can do for your legs. Uphill running is great for virtually all the muscles in your legs especially the quadriceps, calves, hamstrings and glutes. By building your leg muscles, hill running is also great for improved endurance and speed as well.

One of the many exercises available for incorporating hills into a running program are hill repeats. Hill repeats are a great method of building strength, improving speed, and creating confidence in your running abilities. While it may be preferable to find a hilly trail or road for a more varied workout, hill repeats are the best option if you are from an area that is lacking natural inclines in the landscape.

As with any other kind of exercise, it is important to take it easy in the beginning if you have never done any type of hill workout previously. To do hill repeats, run up the hill fast, recover by coasting or walking down the hill, and then repeating the action. As you run uphill it is important that you have proper form. Make sure you lean slightly forward but keep you head straight and chest open. When you are hunched over your lungs breathing capacity can get slightly constricted which will limit your oxygen intake and cause you to tire out faster. Not to mention if you bend over from the waist you are at great risk for injury.

Also to use your energy most efficiently you want to take shorter strides and lift your knees up higher than you normally would. Also make sure you push off your back foot and try to land on the balls of your feet with your heels never touching. When you reach the top of the hill, your legs should feel heavy and your breathing will be quite labored.

When you are first starting out you may want to find a hill that is roughly 30 to 40 yards and run up it starting out at about 75 – 80%. You don't want to go all out too soon as you may just tire yourself out too quickly. When you are on your last couple and you think you have the energy and you want to sprint all out then go for it.

Just be careful to not overdo it or try to force yourself. As you will find out, hill repeats can be pretty exhausting without even having to sprint. While you want to challenge yourself you also want to be safe and not over exhaust yourself and risk injury. If you are able to run up the hill 10 times and you find it to get a bit easier then you can try for 15 – 20 or for slightly larger or steeper hills. Don't be afraid to try and switch things up with this exercise. Remember variety is the key to keep you from getting bored, and it is also good for challenging your muscles.

Although hills come in all different sizes and lengths, doing hill repeats will help to condition your muscles to absorb the shock of running at an incline. While I generally recommend that you walk to catch your breath when going back down you may want to practice running downhill once in a while especially if you plan on running a long distance race such as a 10k or even a marathon. After all when running long races you are very likely to at least some point have to run up and down a hilly landscape.

If you do decide to run downhill the first pointer I want to give is to remain calm. Don't try to sprint as fast you can and don't get over cautious and start to lean back. Just keep calm and sort of go with the flow. You want to lean a little bit forward but not too far forward where you are bending at your waist. You want to make sure that your body is still perpendicular to the ground.

If you lean too far forward you risk injury by putting too much pressure on your body. Not to mention you risk falling flat on your face. I think it is safe to say that this can also cause injury if not just be very painful.

Conversely, you don't want to make the common mistake of leaning backwards either. By leaning backwards you also add stress to your body which will slow you down and even potentially cause injury as well. It is best that you just lean just very slightly forward with your feet always underneath your body.

When running downhill, it also important that you take shorter strides. If you take too long of strides you put a lot of pressure on your knee joints and really risk injury this way. Also be careful not to strike on your heel as this will slow you down and also add stress to your body. You ideally want to land on the middle of your foot and push off as soon as possible.

One last tip when running downhill is to flex your core muscles to help you maintain control and take some of the pressure off your quadriceps as well. Then all you have to do is let the laws of gravity take its course. Please remember that downhill running is generally very hard on your body and should be practiced in moderation and should also be avoided by novices. By applying these rules that I just mentioned however, you should greatly minimize any risk of injury from running downhill.

It shouldn't be too hard for you to see why hill repeats are not only great for conditioning but also for muscle development. However one objection that you may have is that you may have any hills nearby that you can find to run up. Chances are however that if you take the time to look you can more than likely find some sort of hill. Remember that it doesn't necessarily have to be very large.

If anything you can always find a gym and run on a treadmill and just increase the incline. Also many of today's treadmills have workout programs that can simulate hill repeats by periodically changing the incline levels. This may not be the most ideal way for you to do hill repeats, but it certainly is better than nothing. So, regardless of your situation, there should be no excuse for you not to include some sort of hill repeats in your running regiment.

5. High-Intensity Interval Training (HIIT)

Recently named as one of the hottest fitness trends for 2014 by Women's Health magazine, high-intensity interval training (HIIT) involves short, intense bursts of running with active recovery periods of less-intense running or jogging. As all the rage in many running groups and exercise circles across the globe, high-intensity interval training is a super-efficient workout that is ideal for runners with a busy schedule.

Despite the fact that it is such a quick exercise, HIIT has been proven to burn more calories and melt away excess body fat by kicking in the body's natural repair cycle. Even more importantly, HIIT workouts allow runners to preserve their hard-earned muscle mass while still losing weight from fat stores throughout the body.

Without getting too scientific the way it works is that when done properly your body will have a debt of oxygen. In order for your body to replenish oxygen you would need to breathe deeper to take in more oxygen which actually burns calories. If you worked hard enough you can go for hours after your workout and still burn calories. I don't know about you but I think that's pretty damn cool.

One of the best features of high-intensity interval training is that you are in complete control over how fast and for how long you push yourself during the intense bursts of running. After a warm up of around five to ten minutes, HIIT consists of series of near-maximum intensity sprints followed by less-intense recovery intervals of slower running, jogging, or even walking.

The sprint to rest ratio typically is about 1:2. What this means is that if you sprint all out for 20 seconds your recovery or resting period will be for 40 seconds. If you are a novice however you may want to consider a ratio of 1:3 or even 1:4. So if you sprint for 20 seconds you would rest 60 seconds if you are doing the 1:3 ratio and 80 seconds if you are doing the 1:4 ratio.

It is important that you do not cheat your recovery periods. In order to go at 95 – 100% each time you need to make sure that you are adequately rested. Keep in mind that the sprint intervals can be anywhere from 10 seconds to up to 2 minutes. If your intense part is longer than 2 minutes then unless you are in crazy shape you are probably not going hard enough.

The interval times really do not matter otherwise. If you are just beginning I would start with 10 second intervals of going hard followed by 20 – 40 seconds of rest depending on what HIIT ratio you are going by. Then as you get more comfortable you can try sprinting up for 20 – 30 seconds or longer if you think you can. Try to remember to try to switch things up a bit.

Also keep in mind that regardless how long your intervals are this workout should only last you for 15 – 20 minutes. If done properly you should be completely exhausted by that point. By doing HIITs you can get a better workout than a lot of people end up getting and in probably half the time as well.

6. Recovery Runs

Recovery runs are one of the most vital parts of a running program because the human body requires rest from the intensive training that runners put it through. Intense workouts provide the stimulus needed to improve, but recovery runs will help maximize the training benefits reaped from the other different types of running exercises. Some runners refer to these recovery runs as "Zen runs," because they offer the unique opportunity to not focus on burning many calories and instead concentrate on being present in the surroundings.

Since running fast and hard on a daily basis will lead to overtraining as well as increase the risk of experiencing some of the most common running injuries, you will want to add in recovery runs to have a well-balanced running schedule. Recovery runs should be done at an easy pace that can be maintained for a substantial period of time without involving too much exertion.

If you are able to hold a conversation without huffing and puffing while running, you are moving at the ideal steady pace for a recovery run. While these runs are important, always remember that they cannot replace rest days because your body will still need a full day devoted to rest at least once a week.

If you only run a few times a week recovery runs are probably not necessary unless you are doing one right after a hard workout. This is because your legs are getting enough rest with your days off to recover. This is assuming of course you are not doing other exercises with your legs in-between such as squats.

Recovery runs are ideal for runners who run 4-5 times or more a week. You would incorporate them between two extreme workouts. So if you did hill repeats on Monday you would then do a recovery run on Tuesday, and on Wednesday you would do another more intense workout again.

While recovery runs don't necessarily speed up muscle recovery, because they are so light on your leg muscles, they won't impede your recovery either. This means that you will be able to burn more calories by adding more running volume each week without having to worry about hindering your muscles from recovering after an intense running session.

While some runners devote an entire day to recovery running another way to incorporate recovery running is right after an intense running session. This approach has a few different benefits. The first one is that by running lightly after an intense running session, you will prolong your workout, which of course will help you burn more calories. You may not have the energy to do anymore hard running but you may still be able to do some light running as it is nowhere near as exhausting.

Another way this benefits you is that after a hard running session your muscles are in a pre-fatigued condition. When you are running in this state you start to use different muscle fibers that you normally would not use in running. This in turn would help with your running adaptation, which means it will help you build more speed and stamina. This of course is important if you plan on running long distances such as a marathon or a half marathon.

Another way this would help with your long distance running is that it increases your mental toughness. To irk yourself to keep pushing while you are fatigued is not easy to do and if you are not used to running while you are extremely fatigued you will likely never be able to finish a long distance race. By going for a recovery run right after an intense run you can practice on developing the mental fortitude to keep pushing yourself further and further even while you are fatigued.

As you will see this will not be easy to do and if you ever plan on running a marathon or even a half marathon you are going to want to develop your mindset so that you are able to deal with muscle fatigue while you are running. Recovering running is a good way to practice that.

I also want to mention that doing a recovery run in a pre-fatigued state can also be done later on in the day. So for instance a runner may do an intense session in the morning and later on in the afternoon do a recovery run. Your muscles at this point will still be slightly fatigued from the morning run so you would reap the same benefits. Which way you want to approach it is up to you.

As you can see recovery runs plays in an important role in your running sessions if you are looking to reap the maximum benefits from running. Your body was not meant to endure constant intense running sessions on an almost daily basis. So if the previous day you did an intense running session but you don't feel like resting, a recovery run is something you should highly consider doing.

7. Yasso 800s

Yasso 800s are named after the chief running officer at Runner's World magazine, Yasso 800 exercises provide an interesting workout that is often utilized by long-distance runners to predict their marathon time by running equal distances of 800 meters on a track.

Goal times are calculated by taking your desired marathon completion time and converting it from hours and minutes to minutes and seconds per 800m repeat. For example, let's say you want to run a marathon in 3:30. You would then run your 800 meters in 3 minutes 30 seconds.

Although it is commonly a popular form of speed training for marathoners, it can be easily adapted for other training and be incorporated to spice up any dull running program. Since these Yasso 800s follow a rather simple formula, it is usually given the good reputation for being one of the simplest and easiest workouts to remember.

In order to add Yasso 800s into your training program, you will run for 800 meters, recover on a slow jog or walk for the same amount of time it took to run the first 800 meters, and repeat. On the average track, 800 meters is equivalent to two laps around the track and can be converted to around a half-mile in length.

If you are considering a marathon, you will want to start with three or four repetitions in your first week. It is recommended that you continue Yasso 800 workouts once a week, and add one more repetition each week until you reach a grand total of ten.

Even with the proper training, being able to complete ten Yasso 800s in your goal time does not necessarily guarantee that you will be able to finish a full marathon in your desired time. While some runners believe it is a good indicator other runners believe it is a bit fast in predicting your time. This may be due to the fact that it is more for developing speed, and in order to run a marathon you need to develop your aerobic system which the Yasso 800's are not the best for.

However, there is no doubt that completing 10 Yasso 800's is a great challenge. If you are able to complete them, while it may or not give you a great indicator on the time you can complete your marathon, it can still be a somewhat good indication if you have a decent chance to complete a marathon. If anything else it is still a great workout to try whether you are looking to eventually run a marathon, or you just want to add variety to your running routine to prevent boredom.

8. Stair Running

Last but certainly not least, one other running workout you can implement is stair running. Running up stairs can be another great addition to a running program because it comes with the added benefits of building speed, power, endurance, and cardiovascular health. As a great high-intensity sprint workout, stair running is effective at increasing the heart rate and building your leg muscles in great fashion even if only done for 10 to 15 minutes.

Because you are running upwards against gravity you will pump your heart rate at a much faster pace increasing your aerobic system helping with your endurance. At the same time because you are running upwards you are essentially running against gravity which increases your speed and power as well.

In fact when you run up stairs you are using virtually all of your leg muscles including muscles you would not use nearly as much with regular running. Because of this you will burn calories at a much faster rate. In fact you can burn anywhere from 700 to even a 1000 calories in an hour with stair running depending on your body weight. The more you weigh the more calories you will burn as you are pushing more weight up against gravity. This is why stair running can be one of the most effective exercises you can do to lose weight especially if you are obese.

One last benefit to running up the stairs is that you expose your knees and the rest of your legs to less impact when running vertically as opposed to running horizontally. So you are actually less likely to get injured when running up the stairs. However this is not true when going down the stairs so you may want to consider avoiding running down the stairs and walk instead. One other side benefit I should mention is that when you build more muscles in your legs from running up stairs you will also decrease the chance of injury from regular long distance running as well.

Stair running typically consists of running up the stairs, walking down the stairs, resting, and repeating. Many runners decide to run stairs through the bleachers of a stadium, but you may also look for an outdoor stairway or an apartment building that has at least 100 steps to climb. Even stairs from your basement would suffice. Remember if you can't find anywhere close to 100 steps you would just need to do more repetitions.

If you have never done stair workouts before, you should plan to ease in slowly and gradually build up your intensity to risk unnecessary muscle soreness by overdoing it. After building up your endurance by walking up the stairs for your first few workouts, you can begin running after a warm up period of at least five minutes.

On the ascent, actively extend your legs, drive your foot down into the top of the step, pull your toes up toward your shin, and push through your leg with your body weight on the ball of your foot. On the descent, absorb the impact with your glutes and hips rather than your knees to prevent the occurrence of muscle soreness and/or injury.

Typically when running up stairs you will do it in intervals of 1:1 or 1:2 if you are just beginning. Meaning if it takes you 30 seconds to run up a flight of stairs you will then rest for 30 seconds or 60 seconds respectively. If you have several flights of stairs to run up you may want to run up 2 flights of stairs and walk up one as part of your recovery or resting period since it will take you longer to walk up a flight of stairs as opposed to running.

If you only have one large flight of stairs you can walk down the stairs and use that as your recovery period. It's really up to you. Try and experiment with different ways and see which works best for you.

Starting out you may want to only try this for 10 minutes. Remember this is a very intense workout so you may get exhausted very quickly. As you get better, you can try working your way up to 20 or even 30 minutes.

Once you are able to do 30 minutes and you built up your leg muscles and cardiovascular health up more, you can start to challenge yourself other ways as well. You can try running up every other step as long as the stairs aren't too wide of course. You can also carry light dumbbells or wear a weighted belt or vest to increase the intensity and build your leg muscles even more.

As you can see there a lot of different things you can do to keep this exercise exciting as well as challenging. Soon after you start doing stair running it will not take you long to see why this is one of the most effective exercises you can do to lose weight. In fact it may be wise to start out with hill repeats, since this is similar but does not have as steep of an incline as stair running. Once you are able to master hill repeats, then you can start to implement stair running in your running regiment.

Proper nutrition for running

Proper Nutrition for Running

Not only is having a proper diet essential for maintaining good overall health and maximizing the amount of weight lost, but it is also important for enhancing performance while running to burn more calories per workout. Since you will be burning around 100 calories for each mile that you run, it goes without saying that you will need to have the nutrition needed to fuel those miles and make sure your muscles can work efficiently.

While many runners make the mistake of relying on energy bars and packaged nutrient-enhanced foods, proper running nutrition necessitates real fruits, vegetables, lean meats, and whole grains. In order to ensure that you are receiving the proper balance between carbs, fats, and protein, read on to learn the basic nutritional requirements for getting the best weight loss, performance, and endurance out of your body.

Protein

One of the most common diet mistakes for runners is not getting enough protein within their total caloric intake. After all, most sports nutrition experts suggest that proteins make up around 15 to 20% of runners' total daily caloric intake.

Since it may be difficult to calculate how much protein this actually equates to, a general accepted rule of thumb for long-distance runners is to consume up to 1.5 grams of protein for every kilogram that you weigh. For example, if you weigh 140 pounds or 64 kilograms, it is essential that you incorporate around 96 grams of high-quality and lean protein in your diet on a daily basis.

In order to help maximize weight loss while running, you should concentrate on protein sources that are low in saturated fats and cholesterol. High levels of good proteins can be uncovered in lean meats, fish, low-fat dairy products, whole grains, beans, poultry, eggs, tofu, and nuts. In addition to helping you shed the pounds during your workout, protein is vital for regulating your hormones as well as aiding in both tendon and muscle repair to avoid common running injuries. Furthermore, protein is an essential nutrient that is able to keep you feeling full and satisfied over a longer period of time, which is crucial when you are seeking to lose weight.

Healthy Fats

Although it may seem counterintuitive due to the fact that most of us associate a high-fat diet with packing on unwanted pounds, runners need to have a steady supply of healthy fats in order to replenish the glycogen stores that will be used as a vital source of energy on your next run.

After all, health experts declare that adding more healthy fats to your diet can actually help burn more fat and improve running performance for maintaining an energy balance that is conducive to a high level of physical fitness. That being said, it is imperative that runners are able to distinguish between healthy fats and non-healthy fats to make the wisest nutrition decisions.

Basically, there are two separate groups of fats that can make their way into your diet: saturated and unsaturated. As you might predict, the bad fats that should be eaten extremely sparingly are saturated fats, including the notorious trans fatty acids.

Since saturated fats have a bad reputation for increasing the body's cholesterol levels and clog arteries that can lead to heart disease, it is essential that you avoid saturated fats as much as possible. Saturated fats found in high-fat dairy products, meats, poultry skins, and vegetable fats should be limited to just 5% or less of your daily caloric intake.

Instead of consuming saturated fats, it is recommended that you replace them with unsaturated fats and monounsaturated fats that can actually help lower cholesterol levels to lessen your risks for developing heart disease. These heart-healthy fats can be found in nuts, vegetable oils, avocadoes, olives, sesame seeds, and cold-water fatty fish.

Not only will unsaturated fats be beneficial for good overall health and prevention of certain diseases, but they will also provide the essential fats known as omega-3s. Most experts recommend that runners fill 15 to 20% of their total diet with unsaturated fats to get around 3,000 milligrams of omega-3s daily.

Carbohydrates

While proteins and fats are responsible for many important bodily functions, carbohydrates are able to supply the calories that are essential for energy production while running. In fact, carbs have been proven to provide up to two-thirds of the energy the body needs on a daily basis, including for digestion, breathing, and bodily movements.

For rapid and long-lasting energy, the human body works much more effectively with good carbohydrates than they do with proteins or fats. However, in order to ensure the maximum weight loss and receive the energy you need to endure long distance runs, you need to choose your carbohydrates wisely.

According to their chemical structures, carbohydrates can be classified as simple or complex carbohydrates. As their name implies, simple carbohydrates are simple sugars that are composed of just one or two refined sugars that have little nutritional value and are digested by the body more rapidly.

Simple carbohydrates can be found lurking in table sugar, white flour, milk, honey, chocolate, fruit, cake, molasses, sodas, yogurt, and packaged foods. While simple carbs in fruits are healthy, it is advisable that consumption should be limited to small quantities.

On the other hand, complex carbohydrates are composed of a more complex chemical structure that involves a chain of three or more sugars linked together. Due to their complexity, these carbs take longer for the body to digest, do not raise blood sugar levels as quickly, and act as the body's fuel station for energy production. With high nutritional value for providing fiber, vitamins, and minerals, it is recommended that complex carbs make up around 65% of runner's total calorie intake. Whole grains, unrefined pastas, vegetables, potatoes, legumes, beans, and whole-meal breads are great sources of complex carbohydrates.

Vitamins and Minerals

Despite the fact that vitamins will not assist in the energy making process, they are still an important part of the proper runner's diet that has a profound impact on your running performance and endurance levels for going the extra mile. Although many runners swear by added vitamin supplements, ideally the vitamins should be provided from a healthy and well-balanced diet rather than from a bottle.

Since high-intensity exercise can produce free radicals that damage cells, be sure to integrate vitamins A, C, and E into your diet for antioxidants. These vitamins are easily located within carrots, blueberries, sweet potatoes, bell peppers, spinach, kale, broccoli, oranges, almonds, kiwis, fish, and sunflower oils.

Of course if you find it challenging to consume a lot of your essential vitamins whether from not having time to cook proper meals or you're concerned about the processing of the food potentially killing some of the nutrients, then by all means use added supplements if you like. The most important thing is that you actually consume an adequate amount of vitamins and minerals daily or almost daily.

In terms of minerals, it is extremely important for runners to follow a calcium-rich diet in order to build stronger bones, prevent the development of osteoporosis, and avoid the occurrence of stress fractures or other running injuries. You should be able to consume at least 1,000 to 1,300 milligrams of calcium each day naturally in low-fat dairy products, eggs, beans, and even some calcium-fortified drinks.

Furthermore, runners must intake plenty of iron in their diet to deliver sufficient oxygen to the body's cells and prevent feeling fatigued. While men should strive for 8 milligrams, women need around 18 milligrams of iron daily from natural sources like nuts, lean meats, shrimp, and dark leafy green vegetables.

Water Consumption

Consuming enough water every day is crucial for everyone, but it is even more so for runners who will be sweating more than average during their high-intensity workouts. Unfortunately, most runners tend to be unknowingly dehydrated, so it is important to ensure you have enough water consumption to keep the fluids your body needs to function appropriately.

Staying well-hydrated will enhance your running performance as well as prevent heat-related illnesses that can bog you down with fatigue, headaches, muscle cramping, and even decreased coordination. On the flip side, overhydrating can be the cause of abnormal fluid retention that will cause your blood-salt levels to plummet.

Therefore, sports nutrition experts typically recommended that runners take in four to six ounces of fluid every 20 minutes during their runs. Runners who will be pounding the pavement for faster than eight-minute miles should increase their intake to around six to eight ounces every 20 minutes throughout the run as well.

In addition to water, herbal teas, fruit juices, and sports drinks do count as fluids, but you will want to make sure you are not taking in too many excess calories if you are striving to lose weight. Avoid drinking caffeine, sodas, and alcohol as much as possible because these fluids are normally associated with dehydration instead of hydration.

For those who will be participating in longer workouts in excess of eight or ten miles, it is imperative that you make sure you are well-hydrated for at least two days before the long run. As a general rule of thumb, you can tell you are well-hydrated when you eliminate large amounts of pale urine more than six times daily. During longer runs, you should also make sure that some of your water consumption involves sports drinks to help replace lost sodium and essential electrolytes that are voided in sweat. The electrolytes in sports drinks will be effective at helping your body absorb the fluids much more quickly to avoid dehydration.

Well-Balanced Meals

Overall, the most important tactic for maximizing weight loss and enhancing performance is to maintain a well-balanced diet with proportionate meals each day. For runners, it is highly recommended that your daily diet comprises of roughly 20% healthy unsaturated fats, 20% proteins, and 60% complex carbohydrates.

Make sure that you are consuming a good variety of colorful foods, fruits, and vegetables to avoid the need for vitamin supplements in a pill form. When you are equipped with a proper carb/protein/fat balance, you will have the energy, speed, stamina, and endurance to reach your finish line effectively and safely.

Running Injuries

Five Most Common Running Injuries Explained

If you are an avid runner, the chances are high that you have already or will eventually experience an injury. In fact, the latest research from the American Journal of Sports Medicine unfortunately has shown that between 37% and 56% of runners will experience a running injury each year.

While most runners are used to feeling some lingering aches and soreness after a day's work out, severe running injuries can mean a trip to the doctor and a long break from hitting the pavement. Since understanding a running injury is the most essential key towards reacting with the best treatment, the following is an in-depth guide explaining the most common running injuries, how you can avoid them, and the best ways to recover when one of these issues strikes.

1. Patellofemoral Syndrome: Runner's Knee

Since it has been bestowed with the affectionate nickname of "runner's knee," it is no surprise that patellofemoral syndrome is the single most common injury for runners, which accounts for nearly 20% of all running injuries in a given year. As a general term, runner's knee is used to describe localized pain and stiffness under or around the kneecap.

Since women have more flexible joints and more extreme Q angle from hip to knee, it is more likely for females to fall victim to runner's knee. Women who run a 10-minute mile pace or under are even more at risk because the knee goes through a smaller range of motion at slower speeds.

When you start to feel pain around the kneecap, the best first move is to reduce swelling in the knee by taking anti-inflammatory medications, icing, and resting. While you may still run on it as long as it does not hurt too much, be sure to skip long runs and instead focusing on rebuilding your proper running form. In order to reduce your chances of developing runner's knee, strengthen your quads, glutes, and hamstrings with squats and/or lunges to help keep your patella more stabilized. Also, shorten your stride while running to avoid overextension and keep your pelvis level for proper leg alignment that will prevent the knee from collapsing inward.

2. Achilles Tendinitis

When the large tendon that runs toward the back of the heel and attaches to the calf becomes inflamed or irritated; the result is referred to as Achilles tendinitis. Runners often experience Achilles tendinitis due to repetitive stress placed on the tendon, tighten calf muscles, and/or adding too much distance to a running workout.

Usually, this injury will cause runners to feel moderate to severe pain in the area of the Achilles tendon, especially in the morning and with motion. Treatment for Achilles tendinitis typically includes immobilization, plenty of rest, and icing around the tendon.

Since the Achilles is forced to absorb several times the body weight with every stride, men with additional body weight for a BMI of 25 or higher who run a nine-minute mile or faster are at the highest risk for Achilles tendinitis. The injury is also commonly the result of an increase in mileage and high-intensity hill running workouts that stretch the Achilles more on inclines. Runners can reduce the risk of suffering Achilles tendinitis by strengthening the calf muscles with regular calf stretches that lift the toes back towards your shins.

3. Plantar Fasciitis

As a painful common running injury, plantar fasciitis causes the thick tissue along the bottom of the foot to become severely inflamed and irritated. Generally, runners will report experiencing a sharp pain on the bottom of the foot and adjacent to the heel, which is worst in the morning.

Since plantar fasciitis is an overuse inflammatory condition and the surrounded tissue receives minimal blood flow, the injury tends to hang around for extended periods. In particular, men over 40 have the highest risk for developing plantar fasciitis because the tissue becomes stiffer in males and becomes less elastic with age.

While many runners make the mistake of treating this injury with a pressure massage that will only inflame the foot further, plantar fasciitis requires immediate icing and anti-inflammatory medications for temporary relief. If the heel pain becomes too severe, physicians may also suggest a shot of cortisone in acute cases or provide a night splint to avoid tension overnight. Although consistently stretching the calf muscles is beneficial, it is most essential for runners to prevent plantar fasciitis by purchasing good running shoes that provide sufficient arch support.

4. Medial Tibial Stress Syndrome: Shin Splints

Also commonly referred to as shin splints, medial tibial stress syndrome causes a diffused pain and soreness along the front of the shin towards the inside front of the lower leg. When a runner experiences shin splits, the connective tissue in the posterior tibial tendon that runs into the arch of the foot becomes sore and stiff.

Since the tendon has to work especially hard when a person rolls their feet inward when running to counteract this improper motion, medial tibial stress syndrome is most commonly found in runners who tend to over pronate. Runners who are just beginning a training program and those who run on slanted surfaces are also at increased risk.

Due to the fact that leaving shin splints untreated can result into full-blown stress fractures, it is imperative that runners allow enough time for the tibia to heal with rest, ice, and anti-inflammatory medications for reducing acute pain. However, the most effective treatments will need to take into consideration the running errors or abnormalities that caused the shin splints to develop in the first place.

Individuals with medial tibial stress syndrome should focus on strength exercises for the ankle-stabilization and calf muscles. Some runners will also need to wear specially designed motion-control shoes to correct their gait and over pronation to avoid the occurrence of shin splints again in the future.

5. Iliotibial Band Syndrome

Unbeknownst to most of us, the iliotibial (IT) band consists of fibers that lie outside of the hip, down the thigh, along the knee, and to the top of the shin. When this very thick tendon becomes inflamed as the result of overuse, iliotibal band syndrome (ITBS) results and causes pain on the outside of the knee, especially when running downhill.

With surveys showing that nearly 14% of all runners experienced this pain in the past year, the syndrome is typically caused by weak hips and a knock-kneed running form that consequently leads to increased friction and irritation. While ITBS can be an issue for all individuals who tend to run on slanted surfaces, women with a BMI of 21 or higher who do weekly long runs on hills are at the highest risk.

Since long runs in a hill workout often cause the muscles in the band to become fatigued and strained more than normal, it is essential for individuals with iliotibal band syndrome to get rest and avoid these workouts while recovering. Many runners decide to receive an injection of corticosteroid as a short-term treatment, but stretches and massages can also help loosen the tissue as well as reduce the pain. Since biomechanics is also involved ITBS, strengthening the muscles around the IT band with leg walking and foam rolling are effective methods of preventing the reoccurrence of this common running injury for pain-free workouts.

Top Way to Motivate Yourself to Run

One of the biggest challenges of keeping up with your running routine is to keep yourself motivated on a daily basis. There is no doubt that there are going to be some days that you would rather do just about anything other than run. This is why it is very important to find ways to motivate you, to keep moving forward. Here are some very good ways to give you that mental boost that you will no doubt definitely need on days where you just can't seem to get in the right mindset.

Find Your Why- One of the best motivators you can do is to think about your why. What I mean by this is what made you decide to run in the first place? Of course when faced with this question most people will say something like they want to be healthier, or they want to live longer.

However, you should try and be more specific than this. Why do you want to be healthier? Do you want to have a sexier body? Do you want to improve your health so that you don't get sick as often? Maybe you are doing it so that you have more energy throughout the day and therefore you can accomplish more at work and at home.

The same goes for wanting to live longer. If that is your reason you should ask yourself why you want to live longer. Do you want to see your grandkids grow up? Maybe you want to be able to travel to different parts of the world once you are retired and actually enjoy your retirement with your significant other. Again be specific on what it is you want and why you want it and make sure you write it down.

As you write down your why you also want to think about the pleasure you will get from your why. For example think about how great it will be to be more attractive to members of the opposite sex. Think about how great it will feel to be able to fit your old dress or any other outfit that you really like but outgrew. If you want to see your grandkids grow up think about the great future memories you could potentially have with them.

Whatever it is, as you write them down make sure you also include the benefits that will come with it. Then make sure you read it every day. Simply reminding yourself as to why you are doing what you are doing, will give you that extra mental boost you need to push yourself to meet your running goals.

Join a Race- If you are a competitive person than this may be a great way to keep yourself motivated. In fact if you decide to do a marathon or half marathon, you will no doubt have to train for several weeks beforehand to make sure you are in shape for it.

However, you don't need to do a race this large. Even joining a 5k race would more than suffice. If you decide to race, try and give yourself a realistic goal. Maybe you finishing in the top 3 is simply not doable for you, but what about finishing in the top half? Whatever it is make sure it is a goal that you think you can realistically do. Then make a deal with yourself that if you reach you goal you will reward yourself in some way.

Better yet if you have a friend or someone you are well acquainted with that also likes to run try and get him or her to join the race. Then go ahead and make a bet with that person. Perhaps you want to bet that the winner has to pay the loser 100 dollars, or the loser has to take the winner out for dinner or drinks and pay. Whatever it is, make sure it has some meaning to you.

Forcing yourself in some sort of competition can very easily give yourself the motivation you need to meet your daily or weekly running goals especially if you are competing against a friend. When you just are not motivated mentally you can just think about how hard your friend is likely training to kick your ass and take your money or whatever it is you two bet. I don't know about you, but this will more than motivate me to run my ass off.

Run with a Headset- Let's face it. Sometimes running can get a bit boring. However, listening to your favorite new album on your mp3 player or on your phone can take that boredom away really fast. Not to mention it can help adrenalize you to keep at a good fast pace provided you're not listening to r&b or something really slow.

I remember myself one time when on vacation there was a new album that I really liked and wanted an opportunity to listen to. I only had it available on my smart phone. So what did I do? You guessed it. I ran. I attached my headset to my smartphone and went out for a nice run while listening to a new album from a screamo/rock band I really like. I actually ran through the entire album which made for a very long run. But because I was listening to my music it was still very enjoyable so it never was much of a burden to me.

You can also listen to educational mp3's or podcasts as well. Perhaps you are studying for something for college or you are running some sort of business and want to keep educating yourself to stay on top of your game. However, you may just not be up to just sitting at your computer and reading a pdf file or a regular book as well.

Thankfully in today's world a lot of educational stuff that you can read can also be on a podcast or converted in an mp3 format. So if you know you need to study up on a certain topic, but do not feel like sitting, this would be a great excuse to go out for a run.

This way you will be getting some exercise and studying done at this same time. This may not be the best thing to listen to when going for a more intense running session, but if you are doing a long run at a moderate pace or recovery run, listening to something educational may suit you just fine.

Get a Picture of What You Want to Become – This motivational technique is somewhat similar to the first technique, but is more of a visual approach to it. Essentially you will find an image of what you want to look like and keep the picture for yourself to look at daily. So if you want to look like a hot model in her bikini or that guy with the six pack abs you can find a picture of that and keep it somewhere where you can easily reference to it on a daily basis.

You can either get the image from a magazine or even from the internet. If you find it on the internet you can even download the image to your desktop background if you wish or just print it off. Hell, you can even frame it if you like. Just make sure that it is available for you to look at on a daily basis.

Obtaining a nice physique is one of the reasons why many of us like to run. By looking at a picture every day of our ideal body will program our subconscious mind, so that it remembers why it is we are doing what we are doing.

If your physique isn't quite as important to you, but you want to live longer to spend time with your kids or grandkids, then you can look for a picture with a grandfather or grandmother with his or her grandkids. Some of us seem to respond better when we see an actual visual of what we want so this can be a great motivational technique if this describes you.

Give Yourself an Immediate Reward- While having goals and knowing your why is important for motivation, there will no doubt be times when you need some sort of immediate gratification to keep you going. It is going to take a while for you to reach your long-term goals and knowing that you will not see any rewards until a long time may prevent you from finding motivation to run on certain days. This is especially true when you are not feeling energetic and you're mentally exhausted.

This is where having a short term reward can come to play. It is easy to go for a run when you are in the mood are feeling energetic. It's those days when you don't feel like doing it that is the hard part. This is why you may want to have a mini reward system specifically reserved for the days that you would just rather walk on broken glass on barefoot then go for a run.

You can do this by allowing yourself to have a bowl of your favorite ice cream. Or you can treat yourself to popcorn and a movie. It can be anything you can think of that you enjoy. Even if you reward yourself with a bowl of ice cream and put the calories right back on that you just ran off that is okay.

Remember the goal is to make running a habit and in order to do that it is critical that you run even on those days where you know you are supposed to, but just do not feel like it. Giving in to moments of lack of desire is what keeps many people from forming habits. The good news however is that the more times you fight you lack of desire to run, the easier it gets until it does become habit and automatic.

So if you need to reward yourself with something sweet to get you to run on a certain day then do it. Remember, that many people are not able to combat their mental lethargy successfully, so by not giving in to this; that in and of itself is worthy of a small reward.

Other Workouts to Help with Your Running

As time goes on you may want to look into other exercises you can do to increase variety and to also help you with your running. This section will go into different exercises that you can do that will not only help you get in better shape, but will also help you with your running ability as well. So here are some additional workouts that you can do that can help you with your running game.

Plyometrics- Plyometrics are exercises that focus on a particular muscle by extending that muscle and contracting the muscle in an explosive manner to increase efficiency. Runners are able to use plyometrics to help with running speed, power and explosiveness. Unlike a lot of exercises, plyometrics are not about building more muscles as much as learning to use the muscles that you have more efficiently.

Here are a few common plyometric exercises:

Slalom Jump- This is where you stand with your feet together on one side of a line and jump with your feet together on the other side. Repeat this as much as you can, jumping back and forth without pausing. You may find this to be very difficult and only be able to do 4 reps without pausing. Keep doing several sets and keep trying to improve with each set.

Vertical Jump- This is where you stand with your feet hip width apart and start to bend your knees with your hips extended back. Then you would jump straight up from that position and land in the same spot. Again try to do several reps of these without pause.

Water Pump- To perform this exercise stand on one leg with your other leg extended backwards. If you need to place the extended leg on level surface for balance that is find. Then you would simply do a single squat by bending your knee of the standing leg. Try to do this about 15 -20 times and switch legs.

Toe Taps- Try and find any surface that is about a few feet high. Then simply jump and touch your toes from one of your feet on the surface. Before that foot comes down immediately follow up with touching the surface with your toes from you other foot. Then keep repeating this pattern as long as you can without pause.

Like I mentioned, these are just a few of the plyometric exercises you can do. I am not going to go over any more, as there are so many different plyometric exercises it would require a separate book just to go over a good portion of them. If you want to find more out you can easily google them or look up videos on you tube. This is just to get you introduced to them and what they are about.

One last thing I would like to mention is that if you are just starting to get in shape you may want to first practice doing squats or lunges to reduce risk for injury. Plyometrics can have a high risk of injury if you do not have a lot of strength in your legs and core muscles.

Planks- Many people don't realize it, but having a strong core is very beneficial to runners. Having a stronger core keeps your body more strong and stable which will help put less strain on your back and legs. Of course this can help prevent injuries from happening. Not only does having a strong core help prevent injuries but it also improves your endurance and power as well.

One of the best exercises you can do for your entire core which includes your abs, obliques, glutes and lower back, are planks. In order to do a basic plank you would simply go on your forearms and feet and just hold. You should look like you are about to do a push-up but instead of holding yourself up with your hands, you will be on your forearms instead. Hold this for anywhere from 30 – 60 seconds. This may sound easy but if you never have done this before it can be quite challenging.

If you get good at this you can do some modifications to it to make it more challenging. You can try to do what are referred to as plank jacks. This is where you would hold yourself in a plank position. From there you would extend both of your legs outwards like you were doing jumping jacks except your forearms would remain still. Then you would keep bringing your legs inward and outward for the entire time.

Another modification you can try is what is referred to as the super-man plank. This is where you would extend one arm outward and lift the opposite leg up. For example, if you extended your right arm out you would lift your left leg up at the same time. Then hold this for a few seconds and repeat on the other side. Try to keep doing this for about a minute straight.

Also if you want to focus more on your obliques, you can also do side-planks as well. This is where you would lay straight out on one side holding yourself up with your forearm. For an added challenge you can hold yourself up with your hand. Make sure that your legs are stacked right on top of each other. The only part of your legs that should be touching is your bottom foot and maybe part of your ankle. Then hold this for 30 – 60 seconds and repeat on the other side.

There is also a tough modification for this one as well. When you are holding yourself up with one hand, go ahead and take your free arm and extend straight outward over your head. Then bring your top knee up towards your ribs and at the same time take your free arm and bring it down to meet your knee. Hold for a couple of seconds before you bring yourself to your original position and repeat again for as long as you can go. Then of course switch and repeat on the opposite side.

There are many exercises you can do for your core but planks are regarded as one of the best exercises for your core that you could do. Once you start practicing them, it shouldn't take you long to see why. Just by practicing the exercises just mentioned, you should be able to strengthen your core in relatively short period of time. So stop doing those annoying sit-ups and starting building your core muscles with planks. Not only are they more fun, but they are much more effective as well.

Squats or Lunges- If you ever plan to run long distances or try sprinting in your running routines you will no doubt want to have strong legs. Two of the best exercises you can do for your legs are squats and lunges. Both of these exercises target your quadriceps and hamstrings. When you build up these muscles not only do they help you push your body in a forward motion faster helping you with your speed, but they also help protect your knees from all the pressure you place on them helping to prevent injuries.

In order to do a squat you would just stand with your feet straight and planted just over hip width apart. Then bend your knees and buttocks downward until your knees are at a 90 degree angle. Make sure that your knees are not extended past your toes. If they are, you are leaning too far forward. Then slowly lift back up and repeat. Of course for added challenge you can use weights to make it more challenging. You may however want to consider a weight belt if you are lifting heavier weights to help stabilize your midsection.

The second exercise you can do for your legs are lunges. Not only do lunges help with your hamstrings and quadriceps but they also help with your buttocks as well. To do lunges you would step forward and bend your front knee at a 90 degree angle. Your hamstring or back of your thigh should be parallel to the ground. Make sure you lower your back leg so that your knee is hovering about an inch above the ground.

Then step back and repeat to the other side. Of course to make this more challenging you can carry dumb bells on each hand or try doing jumping lunges. So instead of stepping back and forth you would do the same motion but while jumping instead. Make sure not to do this however until you build up your leg muscles a bit to help prevent injury.

Back Extension – As mentioned before when I talked about planks I mentioned how important it is to have a strong core. Despite popular belief, your core is not just your abs and oblique's. Your core also includes your lower back as well. So therefore it is important to have a strong lower back to help with body stabilization and running form.

Just like with the rest of your core if you have a weak lower back you put more strain on your leg muscles causing you to fatigue more easily. Not only that but you also put yourself at higher risk for injury.

Fortunately, there is an easy workout to help with your lower back. This is the back extension. Just lie down flat on the floor on your stomach. Then press your pelvis into the floor as you lift up your head, neck and chest. You can keep your hands around the back of your head like you do when you do a traditional sit-up. Hold for about 5 – 7 seconds and then repeat. It is best to do about 10 reps.

Bicep Curls- It may seem odd but believe it or not your biceps can help play a role in your running form as well. When you swing your arms back and forth you are mainly using your bicep muscles so by building your biceps you can strengthen your motions helping with speed and even endurance.

To do a proper bicep curl you would take a dumbbell and bring it up toward your shoulder. Then slowly go down until your arm is fully extended and bring it back up. You can do this sitting down or standing. Remember that by the time you get to your 8th or 9th repetition you should start to feel a struggle. If you are able to do 10 reps without any struggle then you are going too light. I would advise to do 3 sets of 10 reps for each arm.

Triceps Dumbbell Curls- Needless to say if you want to develop strong arms for your running then you are also going to want to train your triceps in addition to your biceps. To do a triceps curl you would take a weight with both hands and hold it up over your head with your arms extended. Make sure your elbows are close to your head.

Next you would slowly lower the weight down behind your head. Go as low as you can. The weight should be right behind your neck area. Then slow lift your arms back up over your head to their original position. Make sure that your elbows remain close to your head and that you try to only use your triceps to lift the weight upward.

Triceps Dips – If you don't have access to dumbbells than here is another very effective way to build your triceps muscles. Try to find two benches or any surfaces that are about the same height and place them parallel to one another. On one side you will place your heels on and the other side you place your palms hands down. Your hands will be about shoulder width apart while your feet would be close together.

Next slowly dip down. Your elbows should be bent at around a 90 degrees angle. You do not want to go down much further than that as you can start to strain your shoulders. Then slowly go back up and repeat. Try to do 15 reps and 3 – 4 sets. You will find out that this is much harder than it looks.

If you want you can add a weight on your lap to make more challenging. Not only is this exercise good for your triceps but it is also helps with your chest, shoulders and even core muscles as well.

Yoga- One of the most beneficial exercises in my opinion that runners should do that may get overlooked a lot is practicing yoga. Yoga helps with relaxing and can increase your flexibility which can help you recover from beating your body up from intense running sessions. Also because yoga uses a lot of your other muscles that you do not use in regular running it can help put your body in balance. Not to mention that yoga also helps with your core, hamstrings and hip flexors which helps you with your performance and decreases risk of injury.

During one of your resting days would be the most ideal time to practice a light yoga session. Yoga encompasses a lot of stretching which helps with your recovery. Also a quick yoga session could be a great warm up and cool down as well. Yoga helps with loosening your muscles and also relaxes your body as well as your mind. When you are in a relaxed state and your muscles are not tight you use your energy more efficiently which helps you with your endurance.

Another reason yoga makes a great cool down or warm up is that yoga focus's a lot on controlling your breathing which is regarded as pranayama. When you get good with your breathing techniques from yoga, you increase your oxygen capacity which again helps with your performance and endurance.

Keep in mind that yoga can also be used to increase strength in your core area, glutes, quadriceps and other areas of your body. There is a hybrid like style of yoga that focuses more on building muscle and strength that is referred to as power yoga. This involves a mixture of holding tough poses and combing rapid movements. I would not advise to do power yoga on your day of rest or as a warm up however as it can be pretty intense. This would be a good workout option however, if you are looking for ways to improve your strength and conditioning for running.

However since stretching and recovery is really essential for runners I decided to give you a few regular or beginner yoga poses you can start to implement that can be good to do on your recovery days. I am only giving you a few here as there really are a ton of yoga poses out there.

In fact if you are looking for more beginner yoga poses and the various benefits from yoga you can check out my book Yoga 101: Simple Poses to Calm Your Mind & Energize Your Body. You can download it at amazon. Otherwise you can just either buy a yoga dvd, attend a class, or even look up some poses on youtube as well.

Warrior I- Here is a pose to help strengthen your core, hips and legs. This pose can also help you with balance as well. Just stand with your feet together. Inhale. On your exhale step one of your legs straight back and put your arms straight up over your head. Your front knee should be bent at about a 90 degree angle and your back heel should be just off the ground. Hold this position for 7 – 8 seconds and bring your legs and arms back to your original standing position. Repeat 3 – 4 times and then switch sides.

Downward Dog- This is a good pose to stretch your calves and hamstrings. It even is known to help with any back and shoulder pain as well. To do this pose you would begin on your hands and knees and on an inhale extend your arms out. As you exhale you would then pick your knees off the ground and straighten your legs out. Be careful not to lock them.

Then you would stick your buttocks up in the air. Your head should be right between your arms. Try and get your heels to touch, but if you can't that is fine. Just try to work towards it with practice. Hold for 5-7 breaths and come back to original position. Repeat as desired.

Cobra- This is an easy pose that helps with your back and increases the flexibility in your arms, chest and shoulders. Not to mention that because your chest is open in this pose, when you breathe it is known to help with lung capacity as well.

To do this pose just lie face down with your legs about hip width apart. Rest your elbows to your side and keep your palms face down in front of you. Then slowly on an inhale push off from your hands and lift your head and chest and look forward. Make sure your ribs and pelvis are on the ground. Hold for 5 – 7 breaths. Then on an exhale slowly lower yourself back down. Repeat as desired.

Conclusion

I hope that you found this book to be informative and insightful. Most importantly I hope that this book gives you everything you need to motivate you to go out there and lose weight and stay fit. If you are a novice runner this may seem like a lot of information. But don't let that overwhelm you. If you need to, take it in slowly and learn at a pace that you are comfortable with.

Also please remember that the most important thing that you can do is to go out there and run. Nothing is a substitute for taking action. As time goes by you can slowly start implementing the things that you learned from this book and start including them into your running regiment. Try to review and apply at least one new thing from this book every time or every other time you go out for a run.

One last thing before you go. If you found this book helpful I would greatly appreciate an honest review from you. Your feedback is important to me as it lets me know if I am doing a good job and if there is anything I can improve on. You can review the book on the sales page on amazon.com.

Now go out there and run like the wind. Run your ass off!

Other Recommended Books

Run Yourself Skinny: Lose Weight Fast Without Dieting by Michael Thomas

The Science of Running: How to Find Your Limit and Train to Maximize Your Performance by Steve Magness

The Ultimate Beginner Runners Guide: The Key to Running Inspired by Ryan Robert

Beyond Training: Mastering Endurance, Health & Life by Ben Greenfield

Other Books by Max Fischwell:

Mindfulness 101: Mindfulness Training for Reducing Stress & Achieving Everlasting Happiness by Simply Living in the Moment:

Yoga 101: Simple Yoga Poses to Calm Your Mind & Energize Your Body:

Meditation 101: How Anyone Can Easily Learn to Meditate Even if You Can't Sit Still:

Free Yourself From the Shackles of Clutter: Simple & Easy Methods to Declutter Your Home & Other Vital Aspects of Your Life

Free Yourself From the Shackles of Negative Thinking: Eliminate the 7 Positive Killers and Start Living a Fulfilled Life Now!

www.ingramcontent.com/pod-product-compliance
Lightning Source LLC
Chambersburg PA
CBHW071325310526
45789CB00016B/909